WHAT TO DO IN A
PAEDIATRIC EMERGENCY

WHAT TO DO IN A PAEDIATRIC EMERGENCY

A condensed guide to managing paediatric emergencies based on the recommendations of the Advanced Life Support Group

Ian Higginson
David Montgomery
Phil Munro

BMJ
Publishing
Group

© BMJ Publishing Group 1996

First published in 1996
Second impression 1997
by the BMJ Publishing Group, BMA House, Tavistock Square, London
WC1H 9JR

British Library Cataloguing in Publication Data

A catalogue record for this book is available from the British Library

ISBN 0-7279-1032-9

Typeset, printed and bound in Great Britain by
Latimer Trend & Company Ltd, Plymouth

"To live through an impossible situation, you don't need the reflexes of a Grand Prix driver, the muscles of a Hercules, the mind of an Einstein. You simply need to know what to do."

The Book of Survival
Anthony Greenbank

Contents

1 Introduction

2 Initial assessment of the sick child

4 Basic life support

6 Advanced life support

10 Trauma

14 Burns

17 Choking

18 Cardiac arrhythmias

22 Management of acute severe asthma

24 Stridor

26 Shock

30 Status epilepticus

32 Coma

34 Interhospital transporting

37 Practical procedures

45 Index

Introduction

This guide is a user friendly collection of protocols, procedures, and drug dosages to be used in the management of common paediatric emergencies. It is based on the recommendations of the UK Advanced Life Support Group. The intention is to make important information easily and rapidly accessible, and it is compiled for all the groups of health professionals likely to come into contact with sick children. It is not, in itself, a definitive text, and it is recommended that formal training in Advanced Paediatric Life Support be undertaken.

We are grateful to the paediatric staff at Whangarei Hospital, New Zealand, who supported the initial development of this guide, and to the members of the UK Advanced Life Support Group, particularly Dr Kevin Mackway-Jones, for their support. We are also grateful to Dr Duncan Macrae for his contribution to the section on transporting sick children.

Initial assessment of the sick child

*A*irway and *B*reathing:
- Obstruction?
- Work of breathing – grunting, nasal flaring, recession or indrawing
- Respiratory rate
- Auscultation
- Cyanosis?

*C*irculation:
- Heart rate
- Pulse volume
- Capillary refill
- Skin temperature

*D*isability:
- Posture and tone
- Pupils
- Mental status – the AVPU scale
  - A – Alert
  - V – Responds to verbal stimuli
  - P – Responds to painful stimuli
  - U – Unresponsive

It should be possible to perform this assessment within the first minute. If the child is very sick **CALL FOR HELP**. It is better to call for help early. You can then go on to:

- Initial management
- Initial formal observations: pulse, respiration, BP, temperature, O_2 saturations, BM stix, weight
- Initial investigations
- Definitive management

Paediatric normal values

Age (years)	Resp rate (breaths/min)	Heart rate (beats/min)	Systolic BP (mm Hg)	Blood vol (ml/kg)
<1	30–40	110–160	70–90	85–90
2–5	20–30	95–140	80–100	75–80
5–12	15–20	80–120	90–110	65–70
>12	12–16	60–100	100–120	65–70

Fluid and electrolyte therapy
Intravenous fluid requirements:

Body weight	Fluid requirement per day	Fluid requirement per hour
First 10 kg	100 ml/kg	4 ml/kg
Second 10 kg	50 ml/kg	2 ml/kg
Subsequent kg	20 ml/kg	1 ml/kg

The standard fluid bolus in shock is 20 ml/kg.
Fever increases requirements by 12% for each degree celsius rise.

Daily electrolyte requirements:
Sodium 2–3 mmol/kg/day
Potassium 2–3 mmol/kg/day

Estimating a child's weight
Weight (kg) = 2 (Age + 4) in a child over one year
(See also the chart in the Advanced Life Support section p 6).

Endotracheal tube sizes
Rough guide: Tube diameter = diameter of child's little finger or nostril
Internal diameter (mm) = (Age/4) + 4 in a child over one year
Length (cm) = (Age/2) + 12 for an oral tube
Length (cm) = (Age/2) + 15 for a nasal tube

Basic life support

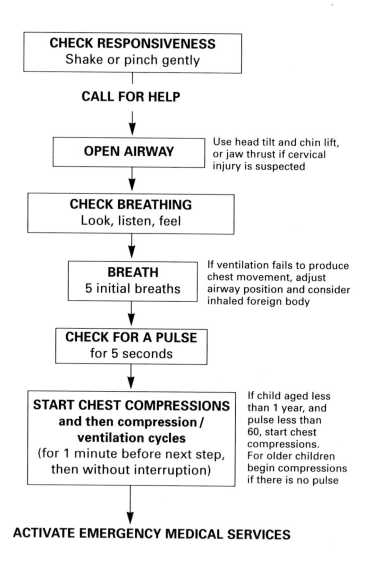

CHECK RESPONSIVENESS
Shake or pinch gently

CALL FOR HELP

OPEN AIRWAY

Use head tilt and chin lift, or jaw thrust if cervical injury is suspected

CHECK BREATHING
Look, listen, feel

BREATH
5 initial breaths

If ventilation fails to produce chest movement, adjust airway position and consider inhaled foreign body

CHECK FOR A PULSE
for 5 seconds

START CHEST COMPRESSIONS
and then compression /
ventilation cycles
(for 1 minute before next step, then without interruption)

If child aged less than 1 year, and pulse less than 60, start chest compressions. For older children begin compressions if there is no pulse

ACTIVATE EMERGENCY MEDICAL SERVICES

4

Summary of basic life support techniques in infants and children

	Infant (<1 year)	Small child (1–8 years)	Larger child
*A*irway position	Neutral	Sniffing	Sniffing
*B*reathing	Mouth to mouth and nose	Mouth to mouth	Mouth to mouth
*C*irculation Pulse check	Brachial or femoral	Carotid	Carotid
Chest Compression: Landmark	1 finger breadth below nipple line	2 finger breadths above xiphoid	2 finger breadths above xiphoid
Technique	Encircling or two fingers	One hand	Two hands
Depth (cm)	1·5–2·5	2·5–3·5	4–5
Ratio of chest compressions to ventilations	5:1	5:1	15:2
Compressions per minute	100	100	80

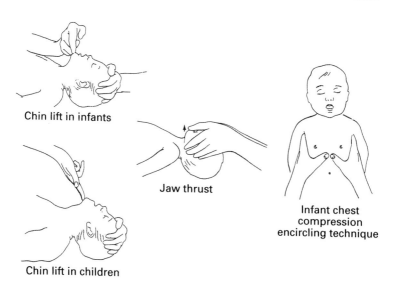

Chin lift in infants

Jaw thrust

Chin lift in children

Infant chest compression encircling technique

Advanced life support

Endotracheal tube

Oral length (cm)	Internal diameter
18–21	7·5–8·0 cuffed
18	7·0 uncuffed
17	6·5
16	6·0
15	5·5
14	5·0
13	4·5
12	4·0
	3·5
10	3·0–3·5

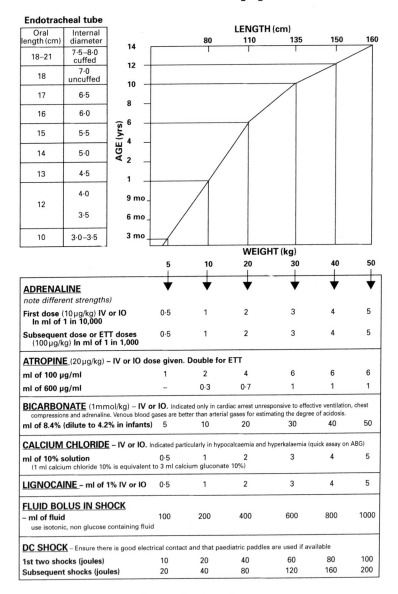

ADRENALINE
note different strengths)

	5	10	20	30	40	50
First dose (10 µg/kg) **IV or IO** In ml of 1 in 10,000	0·5	1	2	3	4	5
Subsequent dose or ETT doses (100 µg/kg) **In ml of 1 in 1,000**	0·5	1	2	3	4	5

ATROPINE (20 µg/kg) – **IV or IO dose given. Double for ETT**

	5	10	20	30	40	50
ml of 100 µg/ml	1	2	4	6	6	6
ml of 600 µg/ml	–	0·3	0·7	1	1	1

BICARBONATE (1 mmol/kg) – **IV or IO**. Indicated only in cardiac arrest unresponsive to effective ventilation, chest compressions and adrenaline. Venous blood gases are better than arterial gases for estimating the degree of acidosis.

	5	10	20	30	40	50
ml of 8.4% (dilute to 4.2% in infants)	5	10	20	30	40	50

CALCIUM CHLORIDE – **IV or IO.** Indicated particularly in hypocalcaemia and hyperkalaemia (quick assay on ABG)

	5	10	20	30	40	50
ml of 10% solution (1 ml calcium chloride 10% is equivalent to 3 ml calcium gluconate 10%)	0·5	1	2	3	4	5

LIGNOCAINE – ml of 1% IV or IO

	5	10	20	30	40	50
	0·5	1	2	3	4	5

FLUID BOLUS IN SHOCK

– ml of fluid use isotonic, non glucose containing fluid	5	10	20	30	40	50
	100	200	400	600	800	1000

DC SHOCK – Ensure there is good electrical contact and that paediatric paddles are used if available

	5	10	20	30	40	50
1st two shocks (joules)	10	20	40	60	80	100
Subsequent shocks (joules)	20	40	80	120	160	200

Resuscitation chart

6

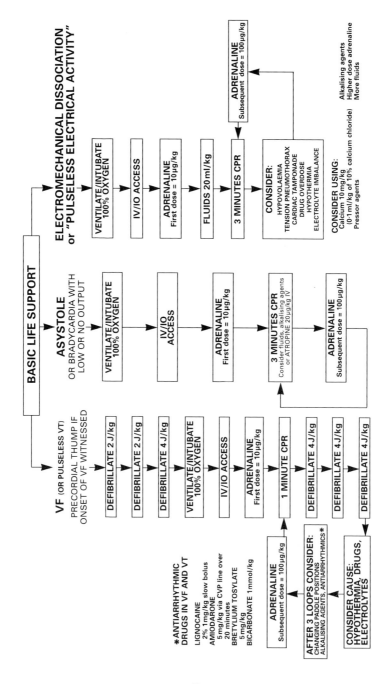

BASIC LIFE SUPPORT

VF (OR PULSELESS VT)
PRECORDIAL THUMP IF ONSET OF VF WITNESSED

- DEFIBRILLATE 2 J/kg
- DEFIBRILLATE 2 J/kg
- DEFIBRILLATE 4 J/kg
- VENTILATE/INTUBATE 100% OXYGEN
- IV/IO ACCESS
- ADRENALINE First dose = 10µg/kg
- 1 MINUTE CPR
- DEFIBRILLATE 4 J/kg
- DEFIBRILLATE 4 J/kg
- DEFIBRILLATE 4 J/kg

ADRENALINE Subsequent dose = 100µg/kg

AFTER 3 LOOPS CONSIDER:
CHANGING PADDLE POSITIONS
ALKALISING AGENTS, ANTIARRHYTHMICS*

CONSIDER CAUSE:
HYPOTHERMIA, DRUGS, ELECTROLYTES

*ANTIARRHYTHMIC DRUGS IN VF AND VT

LIGNOCAINE
2% 1mg/kg slow bolus
AMIODARONE
5 mg/kg via CVP line over 20 minutes
BRETYLIUM TOSYLATE
5 mg/kg
BICARBONATE 1 mmol/kg

ASYSTOLE
OR BRADYCARDIA WITH LOW OR NO OUTPUT

- VENTILATE/INTUBATE 100% OXYGEN
- IV/IO ACCESS
- ADRENALINE First dose = 10µg/kg
- 3 MINUTES CPR
  Consider fluids, alkalising agents or ATROPINE 20µg/kg IV
- ADRENALINE Subsequent dose = 100µg/kg

ELECTROMECHANICAL DISSOCIATION or "PULSELESS ELECTRICAL ACTIVITY"

- VENTILATE/INTUBATE 100% OXYGEN
- IV/IO ACCESS
- ADRENALINE First dose = 10µg/kg
- FLUIDS 20ml/kg
- 3 MINUTES CPR

ADRENALINE Subsequent dose = 100µg/kg

CONSIDER:
HYPOVOLAEMIA
TENSION PNEUMOTHORAX
CARDIAC TAMPONADE
DRUG OVERDOSE
HYPOTHERMIA
ELECTROLYTE IMBALANCE

CONSIDER USING:
Calcium 10mg/kg
(0.1 ml/kg of 10% calcium chloride)
Pressor agents

Alkalising agents
Higher dose adrenaline
More fluids

7

Drug administration during cardiac arrest

INTRAVENOUS ACCESS:
If cannot be established within 90 seconds, go direct to intraosseous access!

- In children any IV access anywhere is effective if drugs are flushed through after administration.

- Central venous access is the best route of administration but should only be attempted by experienced personnel and is relatively contraindicated in trauma patients.

INTRAOSSEOUS ACCESS:
Don't be afraid to try this if necessary – see instructions opposite.

- After giving drugs IO, flush them through. Dilute strong alkalis and hypertonic solutions.

ENDOTRACHEAL ADMINISTRATION:
Any IV or IO access is better than ETT administration

- Only lipid soluble drugs can be used via the ETT – i.e. adrenaline, atropine, lignocaine, bretylium and naloxone.

- Give either (1) via a catheter positioned beyond the end of the ETT tube.
  or (2) by instilling the drug, diluted to 2 ml in N Saline, directly into the tube followed by a flush of 1–5 ml N Saline, thereafter hyperventilating the patient.

Setting up an intraosseous infusion

EQUIPMENT:
Alcohol or Betadine swabs
Intraosseous needle or 16-gauge cannula at least 1·5 cm in length
20 ml syringe with N Saline
Infusion fluid

PROCEDURE:
1. Identify the infusion site. Avoid fractured bones, or limbs with proximal fractures. If possible avoid areas of infected burns or cellulitis.

PROXIMAL TIBIA:
Anteromedial surface, 2–3 cm below the tibial tuberosity.
DISTAL TIBIA:
Proximal to the medial malleolus.
DISTAL FEMUR:
Midline, 2–3 cm above the external condyles.
CONSIDER THE ILIAC CREST

2. Prepare the skin and if necessary use local anaesthetic.
3. Insert the needle through the skin, and perpendicularly/ slightly away from the growth plate into the bone with a screwing motion. There is a give as the marrow cavity is entered.
4. Unscrew the trocar and confirm position by aspirating bone marrow or by flushing with 5–10 ml N Saline.
5. Secure the needle and splint the limb.

Fluids can be infused through an intraosseous needle as through a standard intravenous cannula. If rapid fluid replacement is required, infuse under pressure using a 50 ml syringe. Dilute strong alkalis and hypertonic solutions.
After giving a drug IO – flush it through.

CONTRAINDICATIONS: Ipsilateral fracture. Ipsilateral vascular injury. Osteogenesis imperfecta. Osteoporosis.

COMPLICATIONS: Failure to enter the bone marrow – extravasation or sub-periosteal infusion. Osteomyelitis is rare with short term use. Local infection, skin necrosis, pain, compartment syndrome; fat and bone marrow microemboli all reported.

Trauma

Initial assessment and management

Airway with cervical spine control

Is the airway clear? i.e. speaking or crying. If so give high flow oxygen.

If the airway is not clear give high flow oxygen and perform the following sequential manoeuvres to clear it:

- Chin lift, jaw thrust (Do not tilt head – may have cervical spine fracture)
- Rigid suction
- Oropharyngeal airway (measure from the incisor teeth to angle of jaw – do not use if it makes the child gag).
- Intubation by the most experienced person available
- Needle cricothyroidotomy (see Practical Procedures, p 40)

Immobilise the neck

- In line stabilisation with hands until:
  1 Hard collar
  2 Blanket roll or sandbags or fluid bags
  3 Tape across head and collar onto a spinal board
- If combative, use a hard collar only

Breathing

Once the airway is clear and the C-spine is immobilised:

Is breathing present and adequate? – if not ventilate using a bag-valve-mask system connected to high flow oxygen, using a tight-fitting face mask – this works best with one person holding the mask and one squeezing the bag.

Intubation may be required

Is the trachea central?
Auscultate in axillae
Respiratory rate
Chest wall stability
Wounds, marks or fractures

Clinical suspicion of tension pneumothorax – do a needle thoracentesis followed by chest drain – do not wait for chest X-ray. These procedures are covered in "Practical Procedures".

Circulation and haemorrhage control

- Stop obvious external haemorrhage with direct pressure and elevation if possible
- Insert two or more large bore IV cannulae and draw blood for FBC, cross-match, glucose and urea and electrolytes; and amylase if required.
- Take a set of arterial blood gases
- Replace fluid as follows:

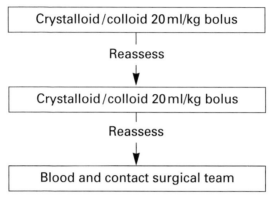

- If you cannot establish IV access get intraosseous access or perform a saphenous cutdown, (See Practical Procedures p 43). Avoid attempting central venous cannulation in shocked children.
- If the patient is shocked and intoxicated, has reduced consciousness, or is otherwise difficult to assess he or she should have intra-abdominal haemorrhage excluded. Diagnostic peritoneal lavage should be performed by the surgeon who will perform any necessary operation.

Disability (neurological status)

Rapid assessment
1 A – Alert
   V – Responds to verbal stimuli
   P – Responds to painful stimuli
   U – Unresponsive
2 Pupils
3 Children's coma scale (see section on Coma, p 33)

Exposure

Completely undress the child but cover with blankets as soon as all necessary procedures and examination are completed.

X-rays
1 Lateral cervical spine (pull arms gently so C7/T1 can be seen)
2 Chest X-ray
3 Pelvis X-ray

Nasogastric tube
Gastric dilation is very common in traumatised children. Pass orally if you are worried about basal skull fracture.

Urinary catheter
Required if the child is unconscious or shocked or has an abdominal injury. Do not attempt if you are suspicious of urethral injury.

Analgesia
Severe pain should be relieved as soon as possible.
The presence of a head injury is not an absolute contraindication provided airway and breathing are closely monitored.

Intravenous morphine is the drug of choice

0·1 mg/kg in an infant or 0·2 mg/kg in the older child. Give the calculated dose in small increments until the pain is relieved
  Never give morphine IM in trauma
  Always record time and dose given
  Can be reversed rapidly with naloxone if required
  Femoral nerve block can be used for shaft of femur fractures
  (see Practical Procedures, p 37)

Tetanus
Immunisation may be required

Arterial blood gases
All patients with breathing problems should have ABGs measured as early as possible and repeated if there is any change in clinical condition or if ventilation is instituted.

Prioritising in trauma

Clear airway
  Protect C-spine
    BEFORE
    Assessing and treating breathing
      BEFORE
      Treating haemorrhage – may require laparotomy/
      thoracotomy to control haemorrhage
        BEFORE
        Treating head injury
          BEFORE
          Treating minor or extremity injury

After **ABCDE** *satisfactory* and *stable*
- Complete head to toe examination, including front and back
- Complete X-rays
- Complete investigations
- Reassess ABCD
- Transfer or refer for definitive care

If there is any deterioration at any stage reassess ABCD

Burns

Don't panic when faced with a burned child. Adhere to the basic principles of resuscitation

Airway and cervical spine

The airway is in danger if:

Burns to face, mouth, or neck
Any suspicion of inhalation injury
Severe smoke exposure in confined space
Soot in mouth or nose
Soot in sputum
Wheeze or stridor

Any of the above should warn that intubation and ventilation may be required urgently – **CALL FOR HELP** – the child may deteriorate rapidly so *do not delay intubation* if the airway is at risk.

Immobilise the cervical spine if injury is suspected.

Breathing

All patients should be given high flow oxygen.
If breathing is absent or inadequate the child will need intubating.

Circulation

Shock immediately after a burn is due to *other* injuries.
IV access should be obtained rapidly
Preferably through non-burned skin (but you may have no other option)
Use the intraosseous route if intravenous access cannot be obtained

Take blood for Hb, urea and electrolytes, and cross matching.
Take a set of arterial blood gases and request carboxyHb.

Give 20 ml/kg crystalloid bolus initially.

Disability

Reduced consciousness level is due to hypoxia, hypovolaemia, and head injury until each is excluded sequentially.

Exposure

Get all clothing off and then cover as soon as possible due to risk of hypothermia during assessment.

Assessing burns

Depth:
  Superficial
    Erythema only
    No blisters
    Do *not* count in % burn
  Partial thickness
    Usually blistered
    Skin pink or mottled
  Full thickness
    Skin white or charred
    Painless
    Leathery, dry to touch

Surface area
Child's own adducted fingers and palm is approx 1% of his or her body surface area. Use the chart overleaf to estimate the surface area involved.
Complete a burns chart while examining patient. (Remember to examine patient's back and back of limbs.)

Treatment

Analgesia
Severe pain should be treated with intravenous morphine
Dose: 0·1 mg/kg in an infant or 0·2 mg/kg in a child
Give the calculated dose in increments until the pain is
  relieved

Fluids
These can be calculated according to the formula overpage

Other
1 Cool burns with soaks or irrigation (not if >10% and not longer than 5–10 minutes). Once the wounds are cooled, dress with paraffin gauze or clingfilm – no flamazine.
2 Insert a urinary catheter if a major burn – aim for at least 1ml/kg/hour urine output.
3 Burns require tetanus cover.
4 Discuss with burns unit fully and if necessary transfer.

Burns: calculating percentage body surface area and fluid therapy

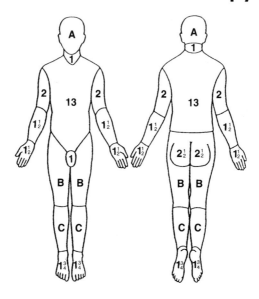

% of total surface area at:

Area indicated	Newborn	1 year	5 years	10 years	15 years
A	9·5	8·5	6·5	5·5	4·5
B	2·75	3·25	4	4·5	4·5
C	2·5	2·5	2·75	3	3·25

Fluid therapy

1. Therapy for shock if indicated (20 ml/kg crystalloid or colloid)
2. Normal maintenance fluids
3. If burns >10% the child will require *additional fluids* (usually 4% albumin) which can be estimated according to the formula:

Percentage burn × Weight (in kg) × 4 (in ml)

Half of this should be given in the first 8 hours *since the time of the burn*. The rest will be given over the next 16 hours.

Choking

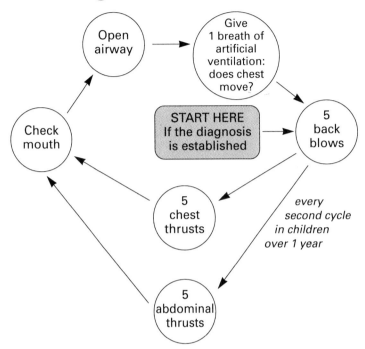

Do not perform blind finger sweeps

Back blows are delivered between the shoulder blades. The child's head should be lower than the abdomen.

Chest thrusts are similar to chest compressions except they are more vigorous but with a slower rhythm. They should be performed at a rate of one every 3 seconds. Lay the child on his or her back, if possible head down along the knee.

Abdominal thrusts can be performed in children over a year of age. Use the Heimlich manoeuvre in conscious children or lay the unconscious child on his or her back. Direct the thrusts upwards towards the diaphragm.

CONTINUE THE CIRCUITS UNTIL THE FOREIGN BODY IS CLEARED.

Cricothyroidotomy is described in the Practical Procedures section, p 40.

Cardiac arrhythmias
Management of supraventricular tachycardia

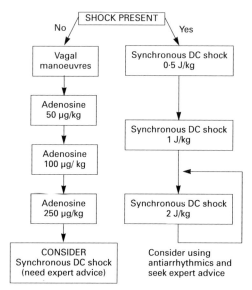

IF IN DOUBT ABOUT ANTIARRHYTHMIC DRUGS AND THEIR USE, SEEK EXPERT ADVICE AND READ THE DATA SHEETS

Adenosine: Give as a quick push via a large peripheral or central vein. Contraindicated in atrial fibrillation with accessory pathways, with some forms of heart block, and in asthma.
Children find the side effects distressing and should be warned about them prior to administration.

Verapamil:
<1 year = do not use   5–10 years = 50 µg/kg IV slowly
1–5 years = 15 µg/kg IV slowly   10–15 years = 100 µg/kg IV slowly

Digoxin: 10 µg/kg per dose IM 8-hourly for three doses, then 4 µg/kg IM or orally every 12 hours.

Amiodarone: 5 mg/kg over 20–120 minutes diluted in approx 4 ml/kg 5% dextrose, by a central route if available.

Flecainide: 2 mg/kg over 20 minutes. Useful in refractory Wolf-Parkinson-White tachycardia. Can be arrhythmogenic and is negatively inotropic.

Management of ventricular tachycardia

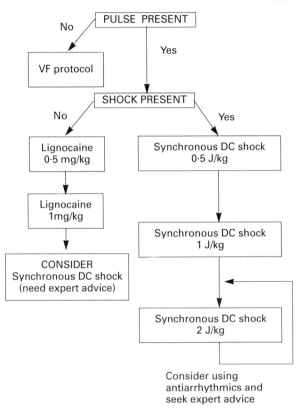

Consider using
antiarrhythmics and
seek expert advice

IF IN DOUBT ABOUT ANTIARRHYTHMIC DRUGS AND THEIR USE, SEEK EXPERT ADVICE AND READ THE DATA SHEETS

Amiodarone: 5 mg/kg over 20–120 minutes diluted in approx 4 ml/kg of 5% dextrose. Give centrally if possible.

Flecainide:
2 mg/kg over 20 minutes. Can be arrhythmogenic and is negatively inotropic.

Phenytoin:
5 mg/kg over 20 minutes. May repeat to a total of 15 mg/kg. Particularly useful in VT due to tricyclic overdose.

Management of wide complex tachycardia

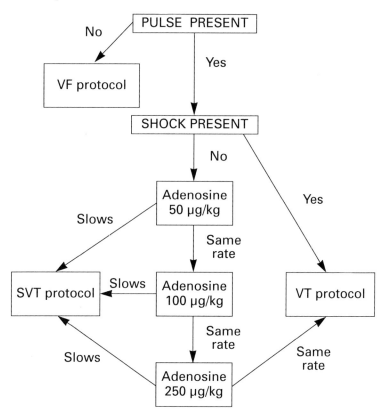

Adenosine:

Give as a quick push via a large peripheral or central vein.

Contraindicated in atrial fibrillation with accessory pathways, with some forms of heart block, and in asthma.

Children find the side effects distressing and should be warned about them prior to administration.

If you are unfamiliar with its use, either seek specialist advice, read the data sheet, or both.

Management of bradycardia

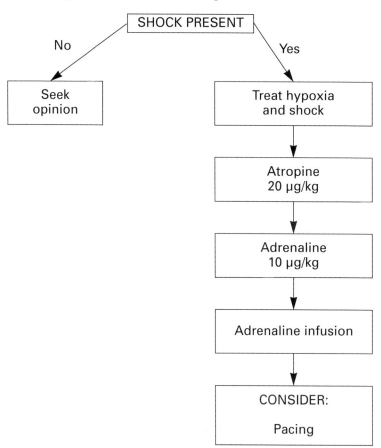

Management of acute severe asthma

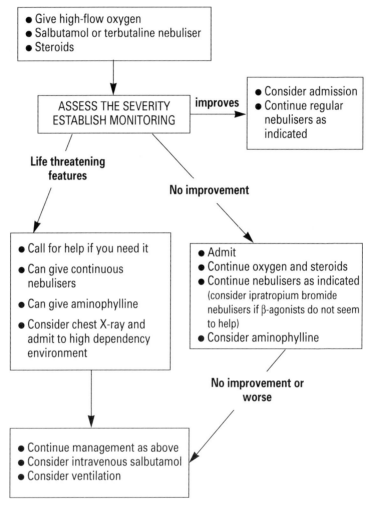

Give high-flow oxygen
Salbutamol or terbutaline nebuliser
Steroids

ASSESS THE SEVERITY
ESTABLISH MONITORING

improves

Consider admission
Continue regular nebulisers as indicated

Life threatening features

No improvement

- Call for help if you need it
- Can give continuous nebulisers
- Can give aminophylline
- Consider chest X-ray and admit to high dependency environment

- Admit
- Continue oxygen and steroids
- Continue nebulisers as indicated (consider ipratropium bromide nebulisers if β-agonists do not seem to help)
- Consider aminophylline

No improvement or worse

- Continue management as above
- Consider intravenous salbutamol
- Consider ventilation

The key to successful management of acute severe asthma is frequent reassessment, aggressive treatment, and plenty of reassurance and explanation.

Judging the severity of asthma:

	Mild/moderate	Severe	Life threatening
Altered level of consciounesss	Nil	Evolving	Yes
Exhaustion	Nil	Evolving	Yes
Cyanosis	Nil	Evolving	Yes
Wheezy	+	+	Silent chest
Retraction	Absent/mild	Present	Obvious
Accessory muscle use	Absent	Present	Obvious
Initial PEFR (% predicted or usual)	>50–60	<50	<33
SaO$_2$ in air			<92%

Monitoring asthma

CLINICAL CRITERIA: Frequent assessment as detailed above is paramount.
PEFRs: Ensure technique is optimal. If possible obtain pre and post nebuliser measurements.
OXIMETRY: Can be very helpful. Consider chest X-ray if poor.

Guide to drug dosages in asthma

NEBULISERS: Give with oxygen, and continue this for at least 15 minutes
SALBUTAMOL ....5 mg as required   } *Half these doses*
IPRATROPIUM BROMIDE ....250 µg every 6 hours   } *in children*
TERBUTALINE ....10 mg as required   } *under 2 years*

STEROIDS:
PREDNISOLONE...........................2 mg/kg daily (max 40 mg)
HYDROCORTISONE ....4 mg/kg every 6 hours. Can give IV or IO.

INTRAVENOUS SALBUTAMOL: use only with advice
LOADING DOSE 5 µg/kg with ECG over 10 minutes
INFUSION 0·6–1 µg/kg/min. This requires continuous ECG monitoring and ICU admission.

AMINOPHYLLINE: use only with advice
LOADING DOSE 5 mg/kg with ECG over 10–30 mins (omit if patient already on theophylline).
INFUSION: Maintenance dose = 1 mg/kg/hour, to a maximum of 20 mg/kg/day
Monitor plasma levels. Reduce dose in liver disease. Interacts with many drugs – consult *BNF.*

Stridor

DIFFERENTIATING CROUP FROM EPIGLOTTITIS

Feature	Croup	Epiglottitis
Aetiology	Mostly Parainfluenza virus	Haemophilus influenzae B
Onset	Over days	Over hours
Preceding coryza	Yes	No
Cough	Severe, barking	Absent or slight
Able to drink	Yes	No
Drooling	No	Yes
Appearance	Unwell	Toxic and ill
Fever	<38.5 C	>38.5 C
Stridor	Harsh, rasping	Soft
Voice	Hoarse	Reluctant to speak, muffled
Wheeze	Often present	Absent
Position	Irritable, active	Sitting forward, neck extended

Remember, atypical cases may occur

Management of acute epiglottitis

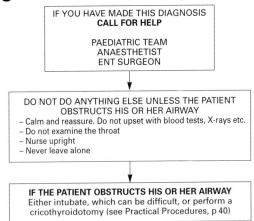

IF YOU HAVE MADE THIS DIAGNOSIS
CALL FOR HELP

PAEDIATRIC TEAM
ANAESTHETIST
ENT SURGEON

↓

DO NOT DO ANYTHING ELSE UNLESS THE PATIENT
OBSTRUCTS HIS OR HER AIRWAY
– Calm and reassure. Do not upset with blood tests, X-rays etc.
– Do not examine the throat
– Nurse upright
– Never leave alone

↓

IF THE PATIENT OBSTRUCTS HIS OR HER AIRWAY
Either intubate, which can be difficult, or perform a
cricothyroidotomy (see Practical Procedures, p 40)

Definitive management will include intubation by an anaesthetist, blood culture and epiglottis swabs, intravenous antibiotics, and chemoprophylaxis for household contacts.

24

Management of croup

1 **ADMIT** if there is stridor at rest, transport or phone difficulties, great distance from the hospital, or concerns over the degree of observation the child will receive.

2 **KEEP CALM.** That includes the child, carers, nurses, and doctors.

3 **NURSE** in a warm, humidified room, and in an upright position. Keep hydrated.

4 **TREATMENT:**
There is no evidence that mist therapy helps in hospital. A child in a mist tent is hard to observe.
Steroid therapy is probably justified in all children admitted to hospital with moderate or severe croup. It aids clinical improvement, and reduces the frequency of intubation and length of hospital stay.
DOSE: Budesonide 2 mg nebulised: useful for acute symptoms and may influence need for admission
Dexamethasone 0·6 mg/kg orally, IV or IM or prednisolone 1–2 mg/kg orally, may reduce duration of hospital stay, and likelihood/duration of intubation.
Oxygen therapy should be instituted in children with *clinical* evidence of hypoxia. Do not rely on oxygen saturations. If a child is hypoxic with croup, close monitoring is necessary, and further measures may be necessary, as it is a late and ominous sign. Humidify the oxygen.
Nebulised adrenaline is useful in relieving airway obstruction. The onset is rapid, and the effect lasts about 2 hours. *There is a risk of rebound effect, greatest up until 6 hours.* The dose can be repeated, and should be augmented with steroids. DOSE: 0·5 mg/kg of 1:1000 preparation (max 5 ml – dilute smaller volumes up to 5 ml with N Saline).
Intubation is the last resort and is indicated if there is hypoxia with progressive airway obstruction, fatigue, or worsening hypoxia.

5 **WHERE TO MONITOR:** Admission to a high dependency area is indicated if there is hypoxia, the child is ill enough to require nebulised adrenaline, or if it looks like intubation will be necessary.

6 **WHAT DOES NOT HELP?** Steam inhalation, antibiotics, sedation, blood tests, X-rays.

Differential diagnosis of upper airway obstruction: CROUP – Viral laryngotracheobronchitis, spasmodic croup, bacterial tracheitis
EPIGLOTTITIS
LARYNGEAL FOREIGN BODY
OTHERS – Diphtheria, retropharyngeal abscess, infectious mononucleosis, angioneurotic oedema, hot gas inhalation, laryngomalacia, congenital deformities.

Shock

Shock is a clinical syndrome resulting from acute failure of circulatory function.

Compensated shock: Sympathetic reflexes conserve vital organ function.

Clinical signs are mild agitation or confusion, skin pallor, tachycardia, cold peripheral skin with poor capillary return. The *systolic blood pressure is maintained* but the pulse pressure may be narrowed.

Decompensated shock: Compensatory mechanisms are failing. Anaerobic metabolism occurs. The patient becomes acidotic. Bleeding diathesis may occur.

Clinical signs include a falling blood pressure, very slow capillary return, cold peripheries, acidotic breathing, depressed cerebration, absent urine output.

Common causes of shock in children

HYPOVOLAEMIC; Haemorrhage, diarrhoea and vomiting, burns, peritonitis

DISTRIBUTIVE: Septicaemia, anaphylaxis,

OTHERS: Cardiogenic causes, pulmonary embolism, profound anaemia

General management of shock

CALL FOR HELP

AIRWAY: Maintain a patent and protected airway. In trauma immobilise the neck.

BREATHING: Assess and maintain. Give as near to 100% oxygen as possible.

CIRCULATION: Obtain IV or IO access. If you are having trouble with this see the section on Practical Procedures (p40). Give crystalloid 20 ml/kg immediately. Take blood for full blood count, urea and electrolytes, glucose, crossmatch and culture.

DISABILITY: Assess the patient's conscious level and pupillary responses. The best initial method is the AVPU score.

LOOK FOR THE CAUSE: basic observations include pulse, BP, respiration, temperature, O_2 saturations, BM stix, and weight.

Hypovolaemic shock

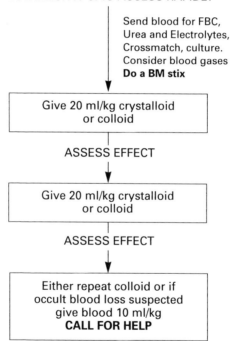

Airway and **B**reathing

Ensure C-spine is stabilised if relevant
Give high-flow O₂

Circulatory Assessment

Pulse rate and peripheral pulses
Blood pressure and pulse pressure
Skin perfusion
Cerebral function

ESTABLISH IV or IO ACCESS RAPIDLY

Send blood for FBC,
Urea and Electrolytes,
Crossmatch, culture.
Consider blood gases
Do a BM stix

Give 20 ml/kg crystalloid
or colloid

ASSESS EFFECT

Give 20 ml/kg crystalloid
or colloid

ASSESS EFFECT

Either repeat colloid or if
occult blood loss suspected
give blood 10 ml/kg
CALL FOR HELP

Remember
- Look for a cause—the most common are detailed above.
- Intubation and ventilation should be considered in a patient who has not responded to 2 fluid boluses

Anaphylactic shock

Stop allergen
Assess **ABC**
Give high-flow O_2

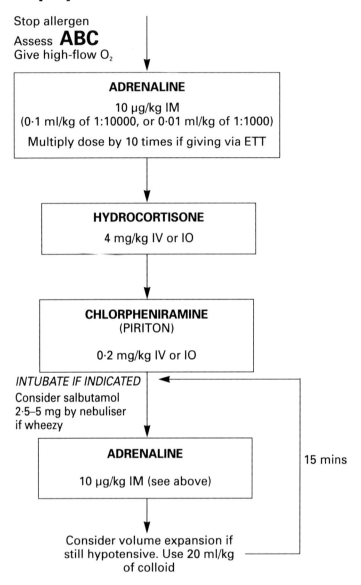

ADRENALINE
10 µg/kg IM
(0·1 ml/kg of 1:10000, or 0·01 ml/kg of 1:1000)
Multiply dose by 10 times if giving via ETT

HYDROCORTISONE
4 mg/kg IV or IO

CHLORPHENIRAMINE
(PIRITON)

0·2 mg/kg IV or IO

INTUBATE IF INDICATED
Consider salbutamol
2·5–5 mg by nebuliser
if wheezy

ADRENALINE

10 µg/kg IM (see above)

15 mins

Consider volume expansion if
still hypotensive. Use 20 ml/kg
of colloid

NB: If adrenaline boluses are not effective, give an adrenaline
infusion (see opposite for dosages).

Septic shock

Make the diagnosis – if sepsis is the most likely cause of shock, contact the paediatric medical team

Airway – ensure patency
Breathing – give high-flow oxygen
Circulation – obtain IV, or IO access if critical. Give 20 ml/kg fluid boluses as required

INITIAL INVESTIGATIONS

BM stix, FBC, U and E, Glucose, calcium, phosphate, *blood culture*. Consider coag. screen and gases

MONITORING

TPR, BP, O_2 saturations, capillary refill, fluid balance, GCS

ANTIBIOTICS: Initially broad spectrum, guided by clinical suspicion.
OTHER DRUGS: (eg) inotropes

FURTHER INVESTIGATION

ONGOING MONITORING

INOTROPE INFUSIONS (SEEK EXPERT ADVICE):

Inotrope	How much inotrope	How to dilute	1 ml per hour equals	Normal dose range
Dopamine	3 × body weight (mg)	50 ml N Saline	1 µg/kg/min	1–10 ml/hour
Dobutamine	3 × body weight (mg)	50 ml N Saline	1 µg/kg/min	1–10 ml/hour
Adrenaline	0.3 × body weight (mg)	50 ml N Saline	0.1 µg/kg/min	1–10 ml/hour
Nor-adrenaline	0.3 × body weight (mg)	50 ml N Saline	0.1 µg/kg/min	1–10 ml/hour

(1) These can be double strength for fluid restricted patients or patients under age 10. The rate is halved if the strength is doubled.
(2) Low dose of dopamine is 2–5 µg/kg/min: increases renal perfusion, no effect of cardiac output. High dose of dopamine is >20 µg/kg/min: increases cardiac output, decreases renal perfusion.
(3) Dobutamine and dopamine are inactivated by alkaline drugs.

Status epilepticus

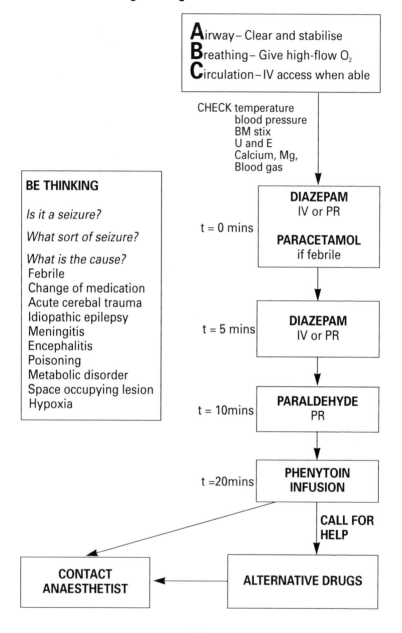

Airway – Clear and stabilise
Breathing – Give high-flow O₂
Circulation – IV access when able

CHECK temperature
blood pressure
BM stix
U and E
Calcium, Mg,
Blood gas

BE THINKING

Is it a seizure?

What sort of seizure?

What is the cause?
Febrile
Change of medication
Acute cerebral trauma
Idiopathic epilepsy
Meningitis
Encephalitis
Poisoning
Metabolic disorder
Space occupying lesion
Hypoxia

t = 0 mins

DIAZEPAM
IV or PR

PARACETAMOL
if febrile

t = 5 mins

DIAZEPAM
IV or PR

t = 10mins

PARALDEHYDE
PR

t =20mins

**PHENYTOIN
INFUSION**

**CALL FOR
HELP**

**CONTACT
ANAESTHETIST**

ALTERNATIVE DRUGS

Guide to drug dosages and use in status epilepticus

PARACETAMOL: 15–20 mg/kg PR

DIAZEPAM: *Rectal:* Age <1 yr use 2·5 mg. Age 1–3 yrs use 5 mg. Age >3 yrs use 10 mg

IV Bolus over 3–5 minutes: Dilute to 10 ml and titrate against effect to max dose of 200–300 μg/kg, or 1 mg per year of age. This dose can be repeated after 10 minutes.

The initial diazepam dose should terminate seizure activity within 10 mins (usually less than 5). The effect lasts a maximum of 1 hour. It is a respiratory depressant, sedative, and can cause hypotension in young infants. MAY INTERACT WITH PHENOBARBITONE TO CAUSE HYPOTENSION AND RESPIRATORY DEPRESSION.

PARALDEHYDE: Rectal: 0·4 ml/kg, made up as a 50:50 solution in arachis/peanut oil, (drawing up the oil first), or as a 10% enema in N Saline.

Paraldehyde takes 10–15 minutes to act. The effect lasts a maximum of 4 hours. This can cause rectal irritation. It causes little respiratory depression. Avoid in liver disease. Plastic syringes can be used, but it is best to do so within a few minutes. Do not use a vial that is discoloured.

PHENYTOIN: IV Infusion: Dose is 15 mg/kg, given over 20 minutes. Dilute in N Saline, usually at 1 mg/ml but can be concentrated to 5 mg/ml if necessary.

Phenytoin should take effect within 10–30 minutes. The half-life is dose dependent. Phenytoin can cause cardiac arrhythmias and hypotension, and ECG and BP monitoring is mandatory. It causes little respiratory depression. DO NOT USE IN CHILDREN ALREADY ON PHENYTOIN UNTIL PLASMA LEVELS ARE KNOWN.

CLONAZEPAM: IV infusion at 10 μg/kg/hr. Causes respiratory depression, hypersalivation, and hypotonia.

VALPROATE: *Oral/rectal/NGT:* Dose is 10–20 mg/kg. Dilute oral suspension 1:1 with water.

IV: Dose is 10 mg/kg. Give over 3–5 mins.

PHENOBARBITONE: IV loading dose is 15 mg/kg given over 10 minutes. Dilute in any standard IV solution. Max dose 750 mg. Phenobarbitone should take effect in 5–20 minutes, and lasts 50–120 hours. It may be effective in patients already on phenobarbitone. MAY INTERACT WITH BENZODIAZEPINES TO CAUSE HYPOTENSION AND RESPIRATORY DEPRESSION.

THIOPENTONE: Induction dose is 2–7 mg/kg IV. Alkaline solution – causes irritation of tissues. This is an anaesthetic agent and should only be used by experienced staff capable of intubation. Other anti-epileptic medication should be continued.

FLUMAZENIL: Give 10 μg/kg stat, then 5 μg/kg at 5 min intervals, repeating up to 3 times. This is used to reverse benzodiazepine induced respiratory depression.

31

Coma

Coma in children is always an emergency – **CALL FOR HELP**

Airway. Establish and maintain an adequate airway
  If there is a history of trauma stabilise the C-spine
Breathing. Give high-flow oxygen.
  Assist ventilation if necessary with bag and mask
Intubation will be needed if ● breathing is inadequate
  ● gag/cough are absent
  ● GCS < 8
  ● There are signs of impending herniation
Circulation. Establish IV access. If there is shock give fluids, otherwise restrict fluids to 2 ml/kg/hr

---

Exclude hypoglycaemia

If present (<3 mmol/l) give
10% glucose 5 ml/kg
Take 10 ml blood and save for diagnostic studies

MONITOR TPR, O_2 saturations, BP fluid balance, GCS

INVESTIGATIONS for FBC, U & E, glucose, calcium, magnesium, phosphate, gases, urine for toxicology?

RAPID GENERAL PHYSICAL ASSESSMENT AND HISTORY
Looking for causes – see opposite

TREAT THE TREATABLE

REASSESS AND DEFINITIVE CARE

Children's coma scale

AGE 4–15		AGE <4 years	
RESPONSE	Score (out of 15)	**RESPONSE**	Score (out of 15)
EYES		**EYES**	
Open spontaneously	4	Open spontaneously	4
Verbal command	3	React to speech	3
Pain	2	React to pain	2
No response	1	No response	1
BEST MOTOR RESPONSE		**BEST MOTOR RESPONSE**	
Obeys verbal command	6	Spontaneous or obeys verbal command	6
Localises pain	5	Localises pain	5
Withdraws from pain	4	Withdraws from pain	4
Abnormal flexion to pain	3	Decorticate posture to pain	3
Extends to pain	2	Decerebrate posture to pain	2
No response	1	No response	1
BEST VERBAL RESPONSE		**BEST VERBAL RESPONSE**	
Orientated	5	Smiles, interacts, follows objects	5
Disorientated	4	*CRYING* / *INTERACTS*	
Inappropriate words	3	Consolable / Inappropriate	4
Incomprehensible sounds	2	Sometimes consolable / Moaning	3
No response	1	Inconsolable / Irritable	2
		No response / No response	1

Some causes of coma in children

HYPOXIC: Ischaemic brain injury following respiratory or circulatory failure, near-drowning

EPILEPTIC SEIZURES

TRAUMA: Intracranial haemorrhage, cerebral oedema or confusion

INFECTIONS: Meningitis, encephalitis, septic shock, cerebral abscess

POISONS: Include psychotropic agents, narcotics, ethanol, salicylates, lead, drugs of abuse

METABOLIC CAUSES: Renal or hepatic failure, Reye's syndrome, hypoglycaemia, diabetic acidosis, hypothermia, Addison's disease, Acute hypo- or hypernatraemia, rare childhood metabolic disorders

HYPERTENSION

VASCULAR LESIONS OR SPACE OCCUPYING LESIONS

INTUSSUSCEPTION

Interhospital transporting

The transporting of critically ill children between hospitals requires a very high standard of preparation and skill on the part of the transport team. Such transfers should ideally be undertaken by a specialised paediatric retrieval team from the tertiary institution accepting the patient.

Stabilisation prior to transporting:

Airway and Breathing: The airway should be secured. If there is any chance of intubation becoming necessary then the child should be intubated prior to transportation. The nasotracheal route is preferred in the absence of a base of skull fracture, nasal obstruction, or significant coagulopathy. The position of the tube must always be confirmed by a chest radiograph, and an arterial blood gas sample should be checked after a period of stabilisation on the transport ventilator.

Circulation: The child should be fully resuscitated. Blood volume deficits must be replaced prior to transportation with colloid or blood. If a low cardiac output persists then inotropic support should be started.

Early management of presenting condition: This may include commencing antibiotics after appropriate specimens have been drawn for culture, stabilisation of fractures, or any other procedures appropriate prior to transfer.

Notes on monitoring:

Essential monitoring required on all transports includes:
   Electrocardiogram
   Non-invasive and possibly invasive blood pressure
   Pulse oximetry
   Electronic temperature monitoring.

End-tidal CO_2 monitoring is desirable, especially in patients with raised ICP

Urine output should be monitored during prolonged transfers

Checklists

Equipment required during transport of critically ill children

Monitors:

    Electrocardiograph

    Blood pressure (cuff and
      ?invasive)

    Pulse oximetry

    Temperature

    End-tidal carbon dioxide

Transport ventilator

Infusion pumps

Resuscitation equipment

Emergency drugs

Portable oxygen supply

Document folder

Maps

Protective clothing

Portable telephone

Pre-departure checklist

Airway: Is the airway secure?

Endotracheal tube: Securely fixed? Correct position? Clear of secretions?

Ventilation: Note respiratory rate or ventilator settings. Blood gas satisfactory?

Oxygen: Requirement for transfer plus at least 30 minutes extra

Circulation: Fully resuscitated?

Major metabolic concerns: Addressed? (eg hypoglycaemia, electrolytes)

Immobilisation: Fractures and if indicated C-spine should be securely immobilised

Monitoring: Is monitoring equipment working? Alarm limits set? Equipment secure?

Drugs/fluids: Sedation/analgesia given?
Infusions running reliably and with adequate volumes for the journey?
All potentially needed drugs and fluids available for journey?

Devices: Nasogastric tube – on free drainage
Chest drains – connected to Heimlich valve and drainage bag?
Urinary catheter?
All devices well secured?

Copies of notes/radiographs

Parents aware of destination and phone number at receiving hospital? Written consent obtained?

Receiving PICU briefed on patient problems, estimated arrival time

Ambulance: patient, staff, equipment loaded securely? Return transport arrangements made?

Practical procedures

Femoral nerve block

EQUIPMENT: Antiseptic solution
1% lignocaine in a 2 ml syringe with a 25G needle
0·5% bupivacaine in a 5–10 ml syringe with a 21G needle

PROCEDURE:
1. Very gently abduct the femur slightly on the affected side
2. Identify the femoral artery and keep one finger on it – the nerve lies immediately lateral to it. Clean the skin
3. Infiltrate the skin with lignocaine and then infiltrate around the nerve with bupivacaine, aspirating frequently to avoid intravascular injection
4. Wait 10–20 minutes before manipulating leg into a splint

Dose of local anaesthetic: Lignocaine 1% 1–2 ml
Bupivacaine 0·5% 10 ml>12 yrs
5 ml 5–12 yrs
1 ml/yr<5 yrs

Needle thoracentesis

MINIMUM EQUIPMENT:
Alcohol or betadine swabs
16 gauge or larger intravenous cannula
20 ml syringe

PROCEDURE:
1. Identify the 2nd intercostal space in the mid-clavicular line
2. Swab the chest wall
3. Attach the syringe to the cannula
4. Insert the cannula at 90 degrees to the chest wall, just above the 3rd rib, aspirating as you go
5. If air is aspirated remove the syringe and needle, leaving the plastic cannula in place
6. Secure the cannula and go on to insert a chest drain

There is a 10–20% chance of causing a pneumothorax in a patient on whom this procedure is attempted, but who does not have a tension pneumothorax. Patients who have had this procedure must have a chest X-ray, and if ventilated will require a chest drain

Chest drain

EQUIPMENT:
Antiseptic solution
1% plain lignocaine
Curved artery forceps
Chest drain (eg 12G infant, 20G child, 28G adolescent)
Large suture (eg O-silk, 2/0 Ethilon)
Underwater seal drain

PROCEDURE:
1. Identify the 4–6th interspace in axilla ("triangle of safety")
2. Clean with antiseptic, drape, and put on gloves
3. Infiltrate with a safe dose of 1% lignocaine down on to the rib and then aim over the upper edge of rib
4. Make a 1·5–2 cm incision along the line of the rib and deepen to the periosteum
5. Gently *blunt dissect* over the top of rib with curved forceps
6. Gently *blunt dissect* through the pleura and open the forceps wide – there may be a hiss of air
7. Insert your little finger into the thorax and sweep around to check your position and to clear adhesions
8. Remove the drain trocar and clamp the tip of the drain with forceps
9. Introduce the drain through the hole aiming towards the scapula and connect to the underwater seal drain
10. The drain should fog with condensation, bubble, oscillate or drain a haemothorax if correctly positioned
11. Secure with a large suture tied round tube, close the incision snugly around the drain, clean, dress with gauze and tape, and use the tape to help secure the tube
12. Obtain a chest X-ray to confirm the position of the drain

Anatomy

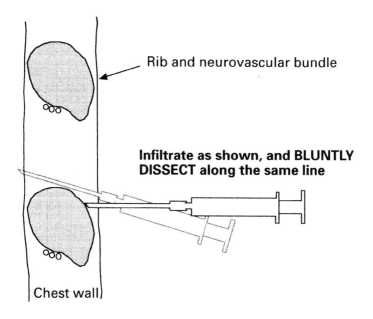

Rib and neurovascular bundle

Infiltrate as shown, and BLUNTLY DISSECT along the same line

Chest wall

Needle cricothyroidotomy

EQUIPMENT

Antiseptic solution or swab

Cricothyroidotomy needle or large IV cannula (16G or larger)

5 or 10 ml syringe

3-way tap or Y connector

Oxygen tubing

Wall oxygen with flowmeter

PROCEDURE:

1. Attach the syringe to the needle
2. Identify the cricothyroid membrane and clean the skin over the area
3. Stabilise the cricothyroid area with your left hand. Extend the neck if there is no risk of C-spine injury
4. Insert the needle through the skin over the cricothyroid membrane at an angle of 45° caudally, aspirating as you go
5. When air is aspirated, gently slide the cannula into trachea – take care not to damage the posterior tracheal wall
6. Remove the needle and recheck air can be aspirated
7. Connect to the oxygen tubing using the 3 way tap or Y connector as shown opposite. You may need a strengthening clip at the join
8. Set the oxygen flow to 1 litre/min per year of age initially. Increase flow as necessary
9. Ventilate by occluding the 3 way tap/Y connector for 1 second, then releasing for 4 seconds. Take care not to overinflate the chest in a very young child
10. Check the neck is not swelling from subcutaneous injection of gas
11. Watch for chest movement, secure the cannula, and arrange for definitive airway – e.g. surgical team to perform tracheostomy

Anatomy

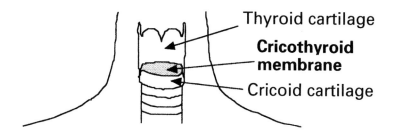

Thyroid cartilage

Cricothyroid membrane

Cricoid cartilage

How to ventilate the patient

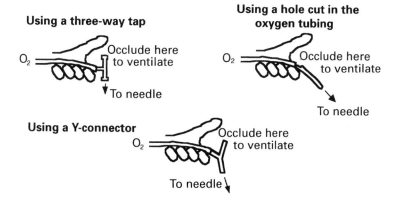

Using a three-way tap

O_2

Occlude here to ventilate

To needle

Using a hole cut in the oxygen tubing

O_2

Occlude here to ventilate

To needle

Using a Y-connector

O_2

Occlude here to ventilate

To needle

Setting up an intraosseous infusion

EQUIPMENT:
Alcohol or betadine swabs
Intraosseous needle or 16 gauge cannula at least 1·5 cm in length
20 ml syringe filled with N Saline
Infusion fluid

PROCEDURE:
1. Identify the infusion site. Avoid fractured bones, or limbs with proximal fractures. If possible avoid areas of infected burns or cellulitis

PROXIMAL TIBIA:	Anteromedial surface, 2–3 cm below the tibial tuberosity
DISTAL TIBIA:	Proximal to the medial malleolus
DISTAL FEMUR:	Midline, 2–3 cm above the external condyles

CONSIDER THE ILIAC CREST
2. Prepare the skin and if necessary use local anaesthetic
3. Insert the needle through the skin, and perpendicularly/ slightly away from the growth plate into the bone with a screwing motion. There is a give as the marrow cavity is entered
4. Unscrew the trocar and confirm position by aspirating bone marrow or by flushing with 5–10 ml N Saline
5. Secure the needle and splint the limb

Fluids can be infused through an intraosseous needle as through a standard intravenous cannula. If rapid fluid replacement is required, infuse under pressure using a 50 ml syringe. Dilute strong alkalis and hypertonic solutions.
After giving a drug IO – flush it through

CONTRAINDICATIONS: Ipsilateral fracture, ipsilateral vascular injury, osteogenesis imperfecta, osteoporosis
COMPLICATIONS: Failure to enter the bone marrow – extravasation or sub-periosteal infusion. Osteomyelitis is rare in short term use. Local infection, skin necrosis, pain, compartment syndrome, fat and bone marrow microemboli all reported

Saphenous vein cutdown

EQUIPMENT:

Alcohol or betadine swabs
Local anaesthetic
Scalpel and curved haemostats
Suture/ligature material
Cannula and infusion fluid

PROCEDURE:

1. Prepare the skin
2. Identify the vein. The saphenous vein runs between half and two fingerbreadths anterior and superior to the medial malleolus, depending on the child's age
3. Anaesthetise the skin if necessary. Make an incision perpendicular to the vein's course
4. Bluntly dissect out the vein, and free a 1–2 cm length
5. Tie off the distal end of the exposed portion – leaving the ties long
6. Pass a tie round the proximal end of the exposed vein
7. Holding the distal tie to stabilise the vein, make a small incision in the vein and cannulate
8. Secure the cannula with the proximal ligature – not too tightly
9. Flush the cannula to ensure patency
10. Secure the cannula with the distal ligature
11. Close the skin incision
12. Secure the cannula to the skin and cover with a sterile dressing

Log rolling children

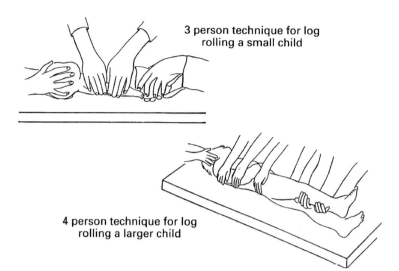

3 person technique for log rolling a small child

4 person technique for log rolling a larger child

Index

acidosis, venous blood gases *v*
  arterial 6
adenosine 18, 20
adrenaline
  advanced life support,
    resuscitation doses 6
  basic life support, doses 7
  bradycardia 21
  endotracheal administration 8
  inotrope infusion 29
  nebulised, croup 25
  shock
    anaphylactic 28
    septic 29
advanced life support,
    resuscitation chart 6
airway
  basic life support 4
  burns 14
  coma 31
  initial assessment 2
  interhospital transporting 34
  oropharyngeal 10
  position 5
  shock 26–9
  status epilepticus 30
  trauma, with cervical spine
    control 10
aminophylline 22
  infusion 23
  loading dose 23
  plasma levels, monitoring 23
amiodarone
  basic life support, ventricular
    fibrillation/tachychardia 7
  supraventricular tachycardia 18
  ventricular tachycardia 19
antiarrhythmic drugs 7
arrhythmias, cardiac 18–21
  bradycardia, management 21
  supraventricular tachycardia,
    management 18
  ventricular tachycardia,
    management 19
  wide complex tachycardia,
    management 20
assessment of the sick child,
    initial 2–3

asthma, acute
  drug dosages, guide 23
  judging the severity 23
  management 22
  monitoring 23
atropine
  advanced life support,
    resuscitation doses 6
  basic life support, asystole 7
  bradycardia 21
auscultation, assessment 2
AVPU scale 2, 11

back blows 17
basic life support 4
  asystole 7
  electromechanical dissociation 7
  pulseless electrical activity 7
  techniques, summary 5
  ventricular fibrillation 7
  ventricular tachycardia,
    pulseless 7
β-agonists 22
bicarbonate
  advanced life support,
    resuscitation doses 6
  basic life support 7
blood
  trauma, replacement 11
  volume, normal values 3
blood gases
  arterial, interhospital
    transporting 34
  arterial, trauma 11–12
    acidosis, estimation 6
blood pressure
  assessment 2
  monitoring 34–5
  normal values 3
BM stix
  assessment 2
  shock
    hypovolaemic 27
    septic 29
  status epilepticus 30
bradycardia, basic life support 7
breathing
  assessment 2

basic life support 5
burns 14
check, basic life support 4
coma 31
  interhospital transporting 34
shock 26–9
status epilepticus 30
trauma 10
bretylium tosylate, ventricular
  fibrillation/tachycardia 7
budenoside, croup 25
bupivacaine, femoral nerve
  block 37
burns 14–16
  ABCDE 14
  assessing 15
  fluid therapy 16
  percentage of total surface
    area 16
  surface area 15
  treatment 15
  urine output 15

calcium chloride, advanced life
    support, resuscitation doses 6
calcium gluconate 6
capillary refill, assessment 2
cardiac arrest, drug
    administration 8
cardiac tamponade 7
central venous cannulation
  cardiac arrest 8
  shocked children 11
cervical spine
  fracture, airway management 10
  immobilisation
    burns 14
    coma 3
  injury suspected, basic life
    support 4
chest compression
  basic life support 4
  landmark, basic life support 5
chest drain 38, 39
children's coma scale 11, 33
child's weight 3
chin lift 4
  children and infants 5
  trauma, cervical spine
    fracture 10
chlorpheniramine, anaphylactic
    shock 28
choking 17
circulation

assessment 2
basic life support 5
burns 14
coma 31
  interhospital transporting 34
shock 26–9
status epilepticus 30
trauma 11
clingfilm 15
clonazepam, intravenous infusion
  31
coma 32–3
cricothyroidectomy 17
  acute epiglottitis 24
croup
  dexamethasone 25
  differentiating from
    epiglottitis 24
  management 25
cyanosis, assessment 2

DC shock, advanced life support 6
dexamethasone, croup 25
diazepam 30
  administration 31
  phenobarbitone interaction 31
digoxin, supraventricular
    tachycardia 18
disability
  assessment 2
  burns 14
  shock 26
  trauma, rapid assessment 11
dobutamine, septic shock 29
dopamine, septic shock 29
drug overdose 7

electric temperature monitoring
    34–5
electrocardiogram 34–5
electrolyte imbalance 7
end-tidal CO_2 monitoring 34–5
endotracheal tube 6
  drug administration 8
  sizes 3
epiglottitis 24
exposure
  burns 14
  trauma 11

femoral nerve block 12, 37
  trauma, analgesia 12
flamazine 15
flecainide 18

46

fluid therapy
  basic life support,
    electromechanical
    dissociation 7
  burns 16
  coma 31
  daily electrolyte requirements 3
  shock 3, 6
    anaphylactic 28
    hypovolaemic 27
  trauma, crystalloid/colloid
    bolus 11
flumazenil 31
foreign body, inhaled
  basic life support 4
  upper airway obstruction,
    differential diagnosis 25

haemorrhage control,
  management 11
heart rate, normal values 3
hydrocortisone 23
  anaphylactic shock 28
hypoglycaemia, coma 31
hypothermia 7
  risk, burns 14
hypovolaemia 7

inotrope
  infusion 29
  interhospital transporting 34
interhospital transporting
  equipment required,
    checklists 35
  monitoring, notes 34
  pre–departure checklist 36
  stabilisation prior to 34
intraosseous access
  burns 14
  trauma 11
intraosseous infusion 9, 42
intravenous access 8
  burns 14
  trauma 11
intubation
  acute epiglottitis 24
  burns 14
  coma 31
  croup 25
  nasotracheal 34
  shock
    anaphylactic 28
    hypovolaemic 27
  trauma 10

ipratropium bromide,
  nebulisers 22–3

jaw thrust 4–5
  trauma, cervical spine
    fracture 10

lignocaine
  advanced life support,
    resuscitation doses 6
  basic life support, ventricular
    fibrillation/tachycardia
    doses 7
  chest drain 38
  femoral nerve block 34
  ventricular tachycardia 19
log rolling children 44

morphine
  burns, dose 15
  trauma, intravenous 12

naloxone 12
nasogastric tube, trauma 12
neck, in line stabilisation 10
needle cricothyroidotomy 10, 40,
  41
needle thoracentesis 10, 37
noradrenaline, septic shock 29

O$_2$ saturation, assessment 2
obstruction, assessment 2
oxygen
  croup 25
  high-flow
    anaphylactic shock 28
    asthma 22
    burns 14
    coma 31

pacing, bradycardia 21
paediatric normal values 3
paracetamol 30,31
paraffin gauze 15
paraldehyde 30
  rectal administration 31
peak expiratory flow rate (PEFR)
  23
peritoneal lavage 11
phenobarbitone 31
phenytoin
  infusion 30,31
  ventricular tachycardia 19
piriton see chlorpheniramine

47

pneumothorax 37
　tension 7, 10
potassium, daily requirements 3
precordial thump 7
prednisolone 23
　croup 25
pulse
　assessment 2
　basic life support 4
　　check 5
　volume, assessment 2
pulse oximetry 22
　interhospital transporting 34–5
pupils
　assessment 2
　trauma, neurological status 11

respiration, assessment 2
respiratory rate 2, 3
rigid suction 10

salbutamol 22, 23
saphenous cutdown, trauma 11,
　43
shock 26–9
　anaphylactic 28
　common causes 26
　compensated 26
　decompensated 26
　hypovolaemic 27
　management 26
　septic 29
skin temperature, assessment 2
sodium, daily requirements 3
status epilepticus 30–1
steroids
　asthma 22

croup 25
stridor 24–5

terbutaline, nebuliser 22–3
tetanus
　cover, burns 15
　trauma 12
thiopentone 31
thrusts 17
transport ventilator 35
trauma
　assessment 10–13
　head injury, analgesia 12
　management 10–13
　prioritising 13

upper airway obstruction,
　differential diagnosis 25
urinary catheter, trauma 12
urine output, interhospital
　transporting 34

valproate 31
ventilation, patients 41
verapamil, supraventricular
　tachycardia 18

weight, assessment 2

x ray
　asthma 23
　chest 12
　chest drain position,
　　confirmation 38
　croup 25
　lateral cervical spine 12
　pelvis 12
　trauma 12

Notes

Notes

Notes

Notes